# THE BHS FACTOR

# THE BHS FACTOR

## THE KEY TO BETTER LONGEVITY

Ralph M. Aurigemma MD

iUniverse, Inc.

New York  Lincoln  Shanghai

# THE BHS FACTOR
## THE KEY TO BETTER LONGEVITY

iUniverse books may be ordered through booksellers or by contacting:

iUniverse
2021 Pine Lake Road, Suite 100
Lincoln, NE 68512
www.iuniverse.com
1-800-Authors (1-800-288-4677)

ISBN-13: 978-0-595-40312-7 (pbk)
ISBN-13: 978-0-595-84688-7 (ebk)
ISBN-10: 0-595-40312-3 (pbk)
ISBN-10: 0-595-84688-2 (ebk)

Printed in the United States of America

# CONTENTS

▼

Acknowledgements ........................................................................ vii

Introduction ................................................................................. ix

## SECTION I

Chapter 1:   Expectations like Promises…Were Meant to be
             Broken .........................................................................3

Chapter 2:   Reality Bites….the Bullet .............................................7

Chapter 3:   Keep Hope Alive ......................................................10

Chapter 4:   The Good, the Bad and the Ugly ...............................13

Chapter 5:   Geriatric Syndromes................................................17

Chapter 6:   Balance....................................................................21

Chapter 7:   With Every Wish…There Comes a Curse .................28

## SECTION II

Chapter 8:   "Back to the Future" ................................................35

Chapter 9:   The BHS Factor.......................................................38

   9.1 Health Factor ...................................................................39

   9.2 Lifestyle Factor.................................................................46

   9.3 Behavioral Factor.............................................................51

9.4 Mental Factor ..................................................................... 57

9.5 Spiritual Factor ................................................................. 62

9.6 Social-Economic Factor ...................................................... 66

9.7 Dimensionality Factor ........................................................ 71

Chapter 10:  What just Happened? .............................................. 78

Endnotes .................................................................................. 81

# <u>Acknowledgements</u>

Thank you to everyone who has helped to make this book a reality. A well deserved thank you to my family for their support, my friends for their wisdom, and my patients for their asking. A special thank you to everyone and anyone who has ever contributed to the sciences, medicine, and caring for their fellow man, the silent heroes who give of themselves selflessly everyday for the betterment of all humanity. And finally, thank you, for purchasing this book. I have every confidence that it will serve you well.

# Introduction

This book is dedicated to better health and well-being for everyone who should desire to improve themselves. It is written for the same reason you are reading it: to create better health for all of us. The purpose is simply to introduce a method that can improve our lives now so that we may enjoy better health later. There exists an abundance of evidence to support the realization that we will not only live longer but that we can also live better. This is exciting information that can enrich our lives.

Therefore, the primary aim of this book is to provide you the information necessary to realize this goal. I will not insult you with false hopes or, more importantly, make hysterical promises or unsubstantiated claims that could place you in harm's way. I provide no dramatics or ludicrous and irrational disclaimers. I make no claims of cures for your diseases, natural or otherwise, and you don't need to get "permission" to read this book from anyone. I simply provide you the truth.

As a physician who practices primarily geriatric medicine I have witnessed the consequences of aging first hand and believe that the current generation of seniors holds the key to future geriatric care. In fact, it is my belief; this current aged population will eventually provide potential information to aid future generations' age better. The BHS Factor or Better Health before age Sixty-Five is an attempt to improve the quality of life for the next generation of seniors based on the experiences of seniors today.

It is quite apparent from caring for such patients that functional limitation accelerates the process of aging. There is also every indication to suggest that functional preservation is the key to improving the quality of life we will experience with our newfound longevity. Therefore, the intended mission of this book is simply to relay the message that by increasing our physical and mental function now, we may enhance function in the future. We, as a population, do not need to suffer the same consequences of aging that this generation of elderly is currently experiencing.

The information in this book is based on facts and not that of quacks that are apparently willing to write anything to sell a book. Contrary to authors who are shameless, as well as, baseless in their criticisms of science and its miracles, this book embraces science, what it has provided us in the past and will continue to offer mankind in the future. Therefore, this book is not written to condemn the efforts of those who have dedicated their existence to the betterment of humanity but to celebrate their vision and accomplishments.

My only intention is to provoke the process of thought within you. I hope to stimulate your interest and awareness through the provision of factual information. Information that may allow you to open your minds to the potential possibilities now available to us, as well as, the inevitable limitations this information might hold. The facts are what they are, how we use this information will determine the outcome.

The most successful people I know are those who have kept an open mind to changes occurring around them. No idea was considered stupid, unworthy, or uninspiring. Rather these people incorporated facts and knowledge to the equation and soon what was considered impossible was reality. If this book does nothing else for you, I hope it instills two basic premises, first and foremost to keep an open mind and second to realize the power of knowledge. A closed mind can make us deaf, dumb and blind, while an open-mind can inspire us to be the very best we can be.

Although this book has been written with an overall lighthearted hand, do not mistake the message it carries. It is written in this manner so that you might enjoy the read. However, of greater importance, it is necessary to recognize the potential value of the information offered throughout these pages. What this information specifically offers and how it can be used successfully to implement a strategy that may ultimately benefit us as individuals. Only by utilizing such a process can you realize the impact this material may have on your life. I feel that I personally have benefited greatly from this information and am living an overall healthier life both physically and mentally. I can only hope the same success for all those who choose to read, absorb and implement this philosophy.

Ralph Aurigemma MD

# *Section I*

CHAPTER 1

▼

# EXPECTATIONS LIKE PROMISES...WERE MEANT TO BE BROKEN

This past New Years Eve I resolved to allot a specific amount of time each week to catch-up on some past due reading. For most physicians this suggests the opportunity to review medical journals which have accumulated throughout the year, or rather, over the course of years. The amount of written material that arrives in the mail to a doctors' office on a daily basis can be, at times, quite overwhelming.

Even if one were to exercise extreme discipline, peruse the journals, identify the "must read" articles and throw out the insignificant material. Chances are there would remain at least one if not two; three foot stacks of journals containing articles with topics of personal interest. The material which physicians' somehow convince themselves will make for leisurely reading over the upcoming weekend.

Of course even the best of intentions don't always workout as planned. For instance, in my case, the journals travel in my briefcase for awhile and eventually find their way to the pile of other unread journals in my office at home. It should go without saying that once they have arrived to this point, their journey is complete. There are now better chances that this pile of shaved wood will sprout roots and find a way to recycle itself into a decorative tree rather than actually ever be read by anyone.

By New Years morning it had already become obvious to me that to meet such grand expectations and keep this resolution, I would have to remain diligent in my efforts. So on the morning of June 17, 2005, I took position under the shade of my office's paper tree and began to read the first article from the journal sitting atop of the pile. The article entitled, *The Looming Crisis in Geriatric Care,* had been published in the June 2000 issue of Postgraduate Medicine.

How a five year old journal had managed to find its way to the top of the pile remains a quandary. However it really made no difference at the time since my intention was to read them all eventually. The first sentence of this article stated, "William Butler Yeats wrote that innocence and beauty have only one enemy-time." The next sentence went on to say, "Good health and longevity also have the same enemy-time." The material was obviously outdated.

As a physician providing geriatric care for the elderly over the past eleven years, such seemingly innocent statements have proven to be unsettling. I have come to realize that good health has little or nothing to do with time. I also recognize that time is longevity's friend and not its enemy. In fact, good health is a reflection of improved access to health care, advances in medicine, healthier lifestyles, better health before the age of 65 and a little luck. Perhaps a lot of luck but time definitely has nothing to do with it.

The "Luck Factors" that I refer to recognizes those things which remain out of our control. Things such as being born into a family with an overall solid gene pool, the ability to successfully cross a street without being run down by an oncoming vehicle and a measurable IQ which allows for the basic ability to think logically. Hopefully, you have been afforded the "Luck Factor" in your life. I can assure you that being a member of this club definitely has its benefits. However, the true key to good health and longevity is not based on luck alone, and it is actually within our control. The secret is better health before the age of 65. This is what I refer to as the BHS Factor and what will determine our future success in the aging process.

BHS is, in and of itself, a reflection and result of several factors. Some of these factors, as previously mentioned, are a consequence of nothing more than luck, and remain beyond our control. On the other hand, factors such as personal behaviors and lifestyle choices are well within our command and can directly influence our health and our lives. The premise therefore being that we as individuals can manipulate our health and thereby manage our own destiny. By simply establishing realistic goals and enacting appropriate lifestyle changes we maybe able to take maximum advantage of the BHS Factor. Only then can we possibly begin to realize our expectations of good health and longevity.

I'm sure that this all sounds wonderful and so easy to achieve. Just simply follow the directions on the side of the box and wah-lah instant gratification, better health and longevity for everyone. However, in real life, the finished product rarely lives up to our expectations and unfortunately the same holds true with regard to the process of aging. Nonetheless, most people have high expectations for their elder years.

Based on my most recent discussions with up and coming baby boomers, it would appear that the majority anticipate aging well. To put it another way, they do not have realistic goals or expectations with regard to their future health or longevity. For example, at a recent speaking engagement I had the opportunity to ask the room filled with primarily baby boomers several relatively simple questions. First, I asked how many participants expected to live into their eighties. The response was overwhelming, more than ninety percent of the crowd showed their hands. The next question was how many expected to be in a nursing home when they were eighty or more years old. The response again was overwhelming, not one hand was lifted. Further questions regarding their level of participation in "Lifestyle Factors" such as diet and exercise, compliance with physician visits and medications, avoidance of tobacco and other risky behaviors all produced variable but overall similar lackluster responses. The group's general underlying assumption was quite simply that "things" would somehow manage to take care of themselves.

This is, in fact, a fundamental philosophy which has become innate to the baby boomer generation, the belief that bad things happen, but not to me. Or what has come to be known as the "shit happens" mentality, where basically an antidotal statement, so cleverly displayed on a bumper sticker, has actually become part of our culture. Such attitudes or beliefs can best be summated though the words of Franklin Adams, who once said that philosophy serves as "unintelligible answers to insoluble problems." Therefore, if one considers that baby boomers represent the most educated, healthiest, wealthiest, and overall best kept generation of our times, it should only seem appropriate that such simple logic would serve as the solution. The underlying premise stemming from the generalized belief that anything is possible, everything is doable and that all consequence are reversible entities.

The principle problem associated with such *"che sera sera"* philosophy however is that eventually it produces complacency. We begin to expect certain outcomes instead of actually realizing them through our own personal efforts. This represents exactly where many Americans are today with regard to so many aspects of their lives including their health. Most people expect to age well regardless of how much time and effort are actually dedicated towards achieving this process.

The anticipated longevity, good health and quality of life expected by the baby boomers, has yet to be realized by previous generations. Nonetheless, the presumption is that everything will work out in the end and everything will be just fine. Are such expectations realistic or rather are they like promises, and meant to be broken. The proceeding chapters may help to change such views and shed light on the realities, limitations and potential possibilities of aging.

▼

# CHAPTER 2

# REALITY BITES....THE BULLET

Expectations and realities are obviously not always consistent and no one knows for certain what the future will bring. However, through the utilization of past and present statistical information it may be possible to provide insight into the future. This information will not only enhance current knowledge regarding modern theories on aging but also aid with future processes.

The importance of this is simply that in the future we as individuals will play a more integral and active role in deciding our personal health care. The provision of health care services for the aging population will present a major challenge in the twenty-first century.[1] Quite frankly, there is a high probability that we may not have access to certain health care services because there just won't be enough to go around.

Allow me to put my pessimism aside for a moment and let's review some numbers. From 1950 through the year 2000 the total population of the United States increased from 150 million to 281 million persons.[2] In relative terms the population doubled. This fact alone represents no obvious crisis.

The cause for concern arises when we take into account the inside numbers and what they potentially represent. For instance, the fact that during this same period of time the population of persons aged 65 years and over grew twice as fast and increased from 12 to 35 million strong. In addition, persons aged 75 years and older were moving at a full sprint and actually grew three times as rapidly, increasing from 4 to 17 million.[3] These numbers provide an open window with a clear view into the future. What they represent is apparent, how they will be interpreted however remains to be seen.

The optimist will have you believe that these numbers clearly indicate increased life expectancy. Actual proof that life can be extended, is indeed possible, and now actually a realization, and should be viewed as positive. However, such a claim would carry much more merit if indeed these persons were not only aging but aging well. The unfortunate reality however is that they are not and thus the concern.

Future projections provide an even more unsettling picture. It is anticipated that from 2000 to 2050 the population of persons aged 65 and over will continue to grow more than twice as fast as the total population.[4] In fact this segment of the population will soon represent approximately 23 percent of the total population. This figure is approximately equal to the number of persons who will be age 18 and under.[5] Such demographics are unprecedented in the United States or, for that matter, any other developed country. Although these figures alone represent a future crisis, we have not yet touched on the crux of the issue.

During the nineteen-eighties, Medicare began conducting annual surveys designed to assess functional limitations among the elderly. These studies concentrated on the limitations most closely associated with the process of aging. The indicators used included a person's ability to perform basic activities of daily living or what has come to be known as (ADL's). ADL's include everyday activities such as bathing, dressing, eating, walking, toileting and rising from a bed or a chair. Through 1992 approximately 16% of people aged 65 and over required assistance with at least one of these six basic functions or ADLs. For persons aged 85 years and over 51 percent were found to require assistance with such activities.[6]

Additional studies have also been conducted to measure instrumental activities of daily living (IADL). IADL's include activities which indicate a person's cognitive or mental capabilities, such as shopping and the ability to manage finances. The results were, and remain, even more discouraging, although these activities are considered more difficult, they are relatively routine tasks. Yet, the pattern that is reveled by these studies clearly indicates that increasing age is directly correlated with increasing disability both mentally and physically.

Further, these studies clearly identify that there is a higher level of disability in women than in men at all ages after 65 years of age. During the twentieth century, even though the life expectancy for men increased from 48 to 74 years of age, women were found to have an increase from 51 to 80 years of age. A rather interesting paradox when we consider that women in general tend to live longer than men in spite of worse health and higher rates of disability.[7]

So what does this all mean? Apparently, it makes no difference if *"Women are from Venus and Men from Mars,"* we all appear to be headed in the same direction and destined to arrive at the same place. Although, we are not quite sure of how to go about getting there or in what condition we will arrive. Every indication would suggest it will not be inline with our current expectations that we will not only grow old but be in good condition once we get there. The truth is, although current studies suggest that our chances of living longer have increased decisively, the evidence is quite clear that we will probably arrive in less than stellar condition. So what does this all mean for us and our futures? Quite simply, reality bites…the bullet.

# CHAPTER 3

▼

# KEEP HOPE ALIVE

So if expectations are nothing more than broken promises and reality forces us to bite the bullet, what hope is there? The baby boomers expectation that the golden years will be truly golden possibly represents nothing more than false hope. The facts suggest that reality will present quite a different interpretation of our future health.

Apparently few people recognize that quantity of life and quality of life represent significantly different destinations. That quantity or over abundance in any form or substance is usually detrimental. The "baby boomer" instinctively believes that more is better and therefore little or no thought is given to the potential circumstances associated with the "privilege" of aging.

Yet, in-spite of all this supposed bad news, there is still cause for hope. Further analyses of the previously mentioned surveys conducted by Medicare provide potentially encouraging news. These surveys initially designed to assess the functional limitations associated with aging, clearly reflect a progressive increase in disability after the age of 65 years. However, from 1992 through 2002 the number of persons who were limited in at least one of six ADLs declined from 16 to 14 percent. Although a 2 percent decline may appear insignificant, in reality, it reflects the huge potential associated with early intervention.

These studies clearly demonstrate the benefits of life style change that are being realized by a minority of seniors today. They are the result of medical research that was published during the nineteen-sixties which identified associations between certain lifestyles and specific disease processes. This research correlated the detrimental relationships between sedentary lifestyles and obesity, high fat diets and heart disease, cigarette smoking and lung disease.[8] Who would have thought that anyone was actually listening?

The results, based on statistics, suggest that people were not only listening but responding to these warnings and implementing interventions or lifestyle changes. Since nineteen-sixty, cigarette smoking has decreased 40 percent. During the same period of time the consumption of saturated fats has also decreased 40 percent, while the number of persons over 40 years of age who claim to exercise regularly has increased approximately 30 percent.[9]

Yet, the finding with the greatest potential significance has only recently been fully realized. Studies have shown that when persons over the age of 65 who are exhibiting functional decline participate in physical therapy and rehabilitation, their level of functional improvement is limited. In fact, much of the functional improvement realized during such programs was generally short lived. In addition, any measurable benefits realized through these programs were lost once they were discontinued. On the other hand, when such programs were initiated in persons less than 65 years of age the overall benefits were substantial. Not only were functional limitations found to improve but in many cases they were reversible. Participants less than 65 years of age were also more likely to continue their physical rehabilitation on their own after the programs were discontinued which resulted in sustained improvements.

The fact is quite simply that people who participate in such programs before age 65 have been found to experience less functional decline after age 65. Potentially as a result of this early intervention and the realization of better health before the age of 65 these people were able to maintain these benefits as they aged. This realization, only now being acknowledged, holds the greatest promise for our generation.

The facts clearly suggest that, so called, "early" interventions can actually take place as late as middle age. In other words, a real opportunity exists to postpone or delay the onset of disability through the alteration of ones lifestyle while in their forties and fifties. Such a revelation quite possibly represents the ultimate "second chance" on life.

Through the many innervations of modern medicine and the pharmaceutical industry, we have been given the opportunity to live longer. Now, it is apparent that through personal intervention we will be allowed the opportunity to live better. However, health maintenance or the BHS Factor will require our personal participation and commitment to be successful. Utilizing these strategies presents us with a genuine opportunity to realize not only longer life but more importantly better quality of life as we age. The bottom line is that there is newfound reason to believe that we can be successful in our quest for better health as we age and therefore reason to keep hope alive.

# CHAPTER 4

▼

# THE GOOD, THE BAD
# AND THE UGLY

This chapter is entitled The Good, the Bad and the Ugly with a specific intent. The premise is to evoke hope while limiting frivolous optimism. While the previous chapter may have provided encouragement, the ability to age "well" should be understood to represent a complex, yet fundamental, interaction between medical intervention, nature's hand, and an individuals understanding and willingness to adapt. There are no guarantees to the processes, they are what they are, but more importantly they are what you make of them.

The good news is the realization that we can potentially intervene in our future health. This represents an immense opportunity for us as individuals to change the proposed and reality based expectations associated with aging. Such knowledge should provide us with a sense of empowerment in that we can actually redirect our future and the "normal" associated consequences of aging. It should also alert us to the fact that many of us have much work to do to accomplish such goals.

The bad news is that the "Luck Factor" can at times be beyond our control. As they say, accidents will happen. In addition to accidental occurrences, we also have little, or no say regarding the gene pool we are provided nor the consequences that it may bring. For example, hypercholesterolemia or high cholesterol levels and the eventual consequence of heart disease associated with this condition can now be decreased through medical and pharmaceutical intervention. Many people receiving medical treatment for hypercholesterolemia, have adjusted their diets, are complying with prescribed medications, and have experienced successful results. The bad news is that such intervention, even in the most diligent person, may not always prove successful.

The down right ugly refers to the development of chronic illness as a young adult. A prolonged course of illness such as diabetes, arthritis or heart disease can produce progressive symptoms that actually accelerate the aging process. As a result of these illnesses, millions of Americans have been exposed to and endure, on a daily bases, increased pain and suffering, decreased physical functioning and limitations in activity. Chronic illnesses not only produce increased disability which decrease quality of life but also account for 7 of every 10 Americans who die each year. More than 90 million Americans live with chronic illnesses and 1.7 million people will die this year as a result of such conditions.[10]

In the years that follow, as the population ages at a record pace, the percentage of Americans afflicted with chronic disease will sky rocket. When one considers the fact that the current cost of medical care for people with chronic illnesses account for more than 75% of the nation's 1.4 trillion dollars spent on health care each year, the future healthcare crisis becomes evermore apparent. The United States cannot effectively address escalating healthcare costs without addressing the development of future methods of prevention for such chronic medical conditions.[11]

Persons aged 65 and under are potential victims of such diseases and their associated disabilities. The years of potential life lost as a result of chronic illnesses are immeasurable. Such conditions are among the most prevalent and costly of all health care problems in this country.

On the other hand, they may also be the most preventable. Middle-aged Americans need to make the effort now to prevent these illnesses in the future. Implementing positive lifestyle changes can produce better health before age 65 which in-turn will insure better health after age sixty-five.

Studies have consistently shown that lifestyle changes after the age of 65 were, for the most part, ineffective. The focus, therefore, is to establish better health before 65 years of age, during our forties and fifties, so that it will carry on into our sixties, seventies and eighties. This in-turn represents the essence of the BHS Factor program.

Therefore, if you are a baby boomer and middle aged, it is essential to implement the BHS Factor into your lifestyles now. However, the goal is not to attempt a full blown lifestyle reform on the first day of the program. Ideally rather, a gradual methodical approach should be sought to introduce such change. For example, start by improving your diet by eliminating saturated and, polyunsaturated fats known as trans fats, or by simply improving your comprehension of food package labels. If you don't have a primary care physician, find one and arrange for a physical exam or check-up. If you're watching four hours of television per day change your routine to only include three hours and walk for one hour. Accomplishing anyone of these tasks will represent long sustained improvements to your health.

Although these tasks may seem simple, they represent invaluable opportunities to improve and sustain long term health. They also represent only the tip of the iceberg. However, the overall general idea is to just get started and to stay motivated, start small and think big. Use whatever method of motivation that works for you to accomplish a task and introduce another and so on. In other words, "just do it."

I know of one person in particular who found motivation by associating this process with the family vehicle. When I inquired as to the logic of this analogy, he simply stated that his family depended on him to provide for them. In-turn, he depended on his vehicle to get him to his job that was forty miles away. The vehicle played an instrumental role in allowing him the opportunity to reach his job and thereby be the "bread winner" or provider. Simple minded, yet prophetic if one considers that as a nation, citizens of the United States spend more money and time each year on the maintenance of their vehicles than on the maintenance of their own persons. We as a nation take better care of our "stuff" than we do our most important resource, namely, ourselves.

# CHAPTER 5

▼

# GERIATRIC SYNDROMES

The elderly population as a whole obviously carries a significant burden of illness and disease. As indicated many people by the age of 65 have encountered multiple medical conditions both chronic and acute. These medical conditions include cardiovascular diseases such as hypertension, coronary artery disease, angina, congestive heart failure, myocardial infarctions, and stroke. Diabetes, osteoarthritis, pulmonary diseases, cancer, and renal diseases also fall into these categories. However, it should be understood by this point that these illnesses represent consequences of living and are not necessarily consequences of aging. These conditions can occur at any age and are usually treatable or rather, more importantly, preventable.

It also goes without saying that such disease processes carry significant long term consequences. Although appropriate medical intervention can reduce the stress that these conditions place on a person and slow their further progression, much of the damage initially sustained as a result of such illnesses is usually not reversible. In the time it takes for your body to recognize that something is wrong or experience symptoms of an illness, the initial or acute encounter has come and gone while leaving behind a permanent and lasting effect. In other words, the body's warning system is about as effective as that of your cars warning light. Regardless of how well the condition is managed in the future the damage has already been done. Again, it can not be stressed enough that disease prevention is therefore essential to preservation.

This chapter, however, will focus on what has come to be known as Geriatric Syndromes. These syndromes alone and in combination represent the true consequences of aging. In other words, if aging was considered a disease process, these symptoms would represent the essence of what the physician would be attempting to treat and prevent. Instead, because aging is a normal process, these syndromes have become accepted as normal consequences of the process. Therefore, little or no legitimate research to access why such dysfunctions occur has been aggressively sought. Furthermore, no preventative measures exist and, in fact, few forms of treatment are available.

It is generally accepted and even expected that as a person ages there will be a constellation of events or symptoms that will affect the persons overall well-being in a potentially negative manner. These symptoms or illnesses include constipation, dehydration, generalized pain, urinary incontinence, malnutrition, falls, dementia, pressure ulcers, vision impairment, hearing impairment, depression, and decline in activities of daily living. Such conditions may seem trivial but they are not. These individual symptoms actually feed off of each other and produce geriatric syndromes.

A syndrome by definition represents a constellation or group of symptoms. Geriatric syndromes in a relative manner of speaking are misnomers in that they are produced by individual symptoms or events which in-turn leads to another series of events. In medical terms the occurrence of a progressive negative series of events is referred to as a vicious cycle. For example, an elderly person drinks 4 ounces less fluid per day for three days and becomes mildly dehydrated. Consequently, this person develops constipation from their dehydration which causes the person to eat less food and eventually become mild to moderately malnourished. Such a scenario is regarded as a vicious cycle. One symptom is feeding off of the preceding event to create a negative outcome.

The vicious cycle describe above is not uncommon and without appropriate intervention it is far from complete. If not properly addressed additional scenarios are likely to follow. Malnutrition can lead to fatigue, decreased activity, bed rest, wounds, infection and death. Mild dehydration may produce a urinary tract infection which causes altered mental status that in-turn may lead to a fall and possible hip fracture. A simple bout of constipation can produce an intestinal obstruction and result in a ruptured bowel, a potentially life threatening condition. The sequences of events and potential catastrophic outcome that may result from the initial condition are endless. Be assured that none of these potential scenarios result in a positive outcome. Therefore, what started out as a "trivial" symptom can result in a serious consequence or catastrophic event.

When geriatric syndromes are placed in their proper prospective, the toll of such conditions on the elderly, and to society, becomes more evident. Studies have shown that twenty-five percent of older adults who sustain a hip fracture are dead within one year of such an occurrence. Consider for a moment that there are 30 million falls reported in the United States each year and that 1 percent or 300,000 of these falls result in hip fractures. Now consider the fact that 25 percent of these people will die within the first year of such an occurrence.[12] The math is simple; it amounts to 75,000 predominantly elderly Americans who will die each year as a result of a potentially preventable fall. Based on these numbers alone, one would be justified in considering this a potential epidemic.

In the future such problems will only become compounded as the over 65 year old population doubles. Add to this the population of over 75 year old persons which is expected to triple and suddenly the word epidemic doesn't appear so exaggerated. The purpose of this discussion is therefore to provide awareness to the fact that "trivial" occurrences can and will produce significant consequences. The general perception that these are "trivial" conditions and represent acceptable consequences of aging is not acceptable. Any deviation from the norm should be investigated.

The premise, simply stated, is that as we grow older we should expect the unexpected but we should not accept the unexpected as normal. It should go without saying that if you experience a change in vision, hearing, memory, bowel or bladder continence, balance while walking, etc., you should see a doctor. If your doctor should inform you that these symptoms represent normal consequences of aging and there is nothing that can be done, quite frankly, you need to find another doctor.

# CHAPTER 6

▼

# BALANCE

If it has not yet become apparent the process of aging is not only demanding but quite complicated. In addition, many of the trial and tribulations of the aged and the aging process are mostly taken for granted by society. We are too consumed with our daily lives to give it much thought and then one day it happens, we wakeup and realize we are old. The reality, however, is that most people will not actually be "old" in terms of age. Rather, they feel old as a result of personal neglect. The process of aging, or rather aging well, requires not only work but more importantly our full and undivided attention.

Most of us realize that quantity or excess, in any form, will usually carry with it certain repercussions. So to with the process of aging there are consequences. However, studies are now providing evidence that these effects of aging can be delayed or in some cases eliminated. The goal therefore, is to use this knowledge to prevent what has to this point been accepted as the "unpreventable" consequences of aging and not to grow old but rather arrive there alive and well. To preserve quality of life so that we may enjoy the privilege that comes with extended quantity of life.

Accomplishing these objectives require specific methods and proper prospective. For example, we all have heard of the jogger or runner who was "in great shape" and that suddenly dropped dead. We all have known the muscle bound weight lifter from high school who shows up at the 10 year class reunion 100 pounds overweight and dies before the twentieth class reunion. In the future, we will undoubtedly know a person who lost 100 pounds by eliminating carbohydrates from their diet while feasting on bacon, cheese and pork rinds only to drop dead several years later from an associated disease. The person "addicted to jogging" is subject to the same pitfalls as the habitual "super size me" individual. Excess in any form will usually result in a negative result.

These types of scenarios are quite common and they should not be viewed as negative. Rather, they represent the positive, hope for the average person to supersede the potential consequences associated with aging. If only track stars were living passed the age of 65, I imagine most of the population would have little hope for the future. The reality is that most people become victims of their own intentions. In other words, running five miles per day eventually leads to joint destruction, limited mobility, loss of independence, depression and death, much in the same manner as habitual eating will lead to obesity, decreased mobility, diabetes or heart disease and death. Extremes in behavior produce a lack of balance.

Balance is an important requirement to achieving better health before and after age 65. However, balance means so much more than just a regimen of proper diet and exercise. We have all heard the phrase that knowledge is power, but it is our ability to think and deduce through reasoning that knowledge is converted into power. Knowledge is nothing more than trash when a person does not incorporate the basic instinct of common sense. Much in the same way that a person who insists that holistic medicine will keep them whole is delusional or the person who believes that their cancer will be cured with acupuncture treatments will die, the person who only seeks medical care when they are sick is doomed.

Therefore, it is essential to establish balance in our lives. The best example, of the balance, I am referring to can be clearly seen in an individual who, if identified, would be readily recognized by most readers. This person not only represents perfect balance but is the ideal example of someone who is taking full advantage of the BHS Factor. This is a person who exercises daily, eats a proper diet, drinks plenty of water, and follows safety-first practices. In addition, this individual consumes approximately 50 to 60 vitamin and mineral pills per day, is an avid "juicer", practices yoga and meditation, regularly undergoes acupuncture treatments, and occasionally visits a chiropractor for muscle-skeletal manipulation. He prays religiously, is family oriented, and an active member of his community. He practices routine health maintenance, takes an antihypertensive and a cholesterol lowering medication. He is not following a holistic, alternative or traditional lifestyle, but rather, he is living a "balanced" life. He participates in unproven practices that he feels are helpful and pleasing to him while not denying himself the benefits of proven modern medicine. He obviously is open-minded and this is the essential element that allows him to take full advantage of the options that are available, not only to him, but to all of us. He is the ideal representative of a real world man, a renaissance man, a visionary.

Unfortunately, there are not many people who share this interpretation. Most people will assume this individual just has too much time on his hands. I am aware of both his personal schedule and his work schedule and I can assure you he does not have the time to spare. Rather, he is, not taking, but making the time to fulfill what is important to him. He is creating a lifestyle as apposed to settling for one.

Many people in this country do not take advantage of that which is available to them. They therefore find themselves settling for less than the best. These people are perfectly content remaining uninformed, misinformed or actually ignoring information that is readily available to them. In many cases this occurs as a direct result of bias, prejudices, and in many cases having been brainwashed. Such people are actually willing to deprive themselves of proven scientific methods in a so called effort to "buck" the system. These are the people currently purchasing a recently published book entitled "Natural Cures", by Kevin Trudeau, and making it a best seller.

According to Mr. Trudeau's self publicity, millions of people have supposedly bought his book. Yes, you are reading this correctly. Millions of people have thought nothing of paying thirty dollars for medical advice from a convicted felon. These are the same people who lament when asked for their insurance co-pay at the time of their physician visits.

I must admit that I also plunked down my hard earned cash for a copy of this book. I too needed to know the secrets that "doctors don't want us to know." The reality however is that his book literally says nothing, there are no hidden secrets revealed and there are no cures for ailments. The message is nothing more than that of a rebellious teenager consumed with anti-establishment rhetoric. Quite simply; don't trust government or big business, including pharmaceutical companies, food companies, and even small businesses such as your doctor.

I have even heard Howard Stern, a celebrated raunchy talk show host, who, on the other hand, is usually a quasi-logical and well informed person, state that he was actually "enjoying" the book. You may ask yourself, why it should matter what Howard Stern chooses to think. It matters in that he has millions of listeners who cling to his views and beliefs. No different from the legions of listeners and viewers who tune into the drug abusing, pill popping Rush Limbaugh or the self righteous, phone sex addicted, Bill O'Rielly. The point is simply that the American public is easily influenced and quite willing to accept what such media personalities are selling or dishing out on any given day. My advice is simple, make your own choices! The decisions we make and decide to follow can influence and affect our lives forever. Please don't allow anyone to make such decisions for you! Especially a person such as Kevin Trudeau, a self proclaimed conman who is more than willing to shamelessly misinform the public and sell people false hope in order to fulfill his own agenda.

Mr. Trudeau has no medical training, yet he claims to have a cure for virtually every disease process known to man kind. He tells his audience that physicians and pharmaceutical companies are all crooks and should not be trusted. He says that all medicines are poison and actually instructs people to stop taking their medications, but of course, to first inform their "untrustworthy" physicians. The reason for my continued ranting on this subject represents my frustration with the author's unconscionable bad advice, my point however is simply to trust your ability to make your own decisions. Incorporate the facts and establish a plan based on your understanding of the truth, and you will make the right choices.

We are constantly being subjected to general misconceptions and "urban myths" which are accepted at face value. For example, regardless of the health care and health insurance crisis, there is no shortage of health care providers in this country. In fact, there is currently greater access to health care, in this country, than ever before. In addition, with the advent of new pharmaceuticals designed to prevent and reverse disease rather than just treat illness, the medical community has embraced preventative medicine and the promise which it holds. This availability and new age thinking represents the added advantage previous shorter lived generations lacked. An individual's choice to neglect these options for what are unproven alternatives, or choosing to avoid these options, due to fear of physicians or medications, are just as illogical as accepting your friends prescription medication to treat your headache.

Common sense is a powerful tool that is more often than not underutilized. The world is filled with people who struggle with, do without thinking, or think without doing, personalities. There are the people who refuse to drive a car without wearing a seatbelt but think nothing of riding a motorcycle without a helmet. At the opposite end of the spectrum are the people who procrastinate and over-think their every decision. The individual who, visits a doctor regularly, is eventually prescribed a medication for high blood pressure and after reading the list of side effects decides not to take the medication. Both of the above described behaviors represent scenarios that should be considered reckless and dangerous, with potentially severe consequences. However, I am reasonably confident that a high percentage of people comparing these two circumstances felt that the second person who decided not to take the prescribed medication was justified in their thinking. The reality, however, is that this person is in fact at greater risk of harm than the idiot, without a helmet, on the motorcycle. The truth is that the benefits of taking the pill far outweigh the potential risk or side effects associated with taking the prescribed medication. Comparing the potential risk or consequences associated with not taking the pill versus a person riding a motorcycle without a helmet, the person on the motorcycle's risk of injury is almost negligible.

Changing ones attitude and behavior can be difficult. Every situation needs to be evaluated individually so that a logical choice can be made. Factual information represents the main stay of logic. While mystical thinking, bias, fear and fiction interfere with the decision making process. However, all too often, reasonable people are asked to make desperate choices. These ill and distressed people who are under the influence of unusual and overwhelming stress are placed in a position where they are expected to make life altering medical choices. Their circumstances hinder reasonable decision making abilities, if one considers that these people are usually in a state of denial or anger when such decisions are made, it becomes even more apparent as to why such conclusions are reached. However, my concern is more with the everyday person, who is not under such stress, making everyday choices. What is it that leads such people to make such unacceptable choices?

Why do reasonable people, in many cases highly educated people, subject themselves to unreasonable options? People with relatively easy to treat conditions, which opt for religious intervention, alternative medicine, or vitamins and supplements, as the basis of their treatment and reject the opportunities available to them through conventional medicine. How can one believe that a prayer will be answered for an individual as apposed to God having given another human being the ability to develop a treatment to heal or help thousands upon thousands? How can people have such faith in God as creator and yet not be capable of trusting that which God has created? Miracles come in all shapes and forms and actually are occurring every single day, don't be blind to the obvious. The point is that, although there is usually no harm incorporating alternative therapies into our health care plans', eliminating a proven resource, is foolish.

It is important that we always consider all options and keep an open mind in everything we do. When addressing a medical illness, the rule should be to consider all options! There is little potential for harm through the process of inclusion, while misinformation or inappropriate and reckless exclusion can produce significant consequences. Information produces knowledge and thereby allows us an opportunity to make our own choice. Incorporating logic into this equation, however, allows us the opportunity to make the right choices. These are the essential elements that make up the concept of balance, it is impervious that we recognize and accept them as part of our lives.

# CHAPTER 7

▼

# WITH EVERY WISH…THERE COMES A CURSE

The realization of balance in our lives allows us the opportunity to rationalize and make decisions more clearly and thereby have more control. This process thereby enables us to realize better outcomes based on our ability to make better decisions. This, in and of itself, will effect your life in ways that you may have never thought possible. It will prove effective in your career, finances, how you interact with your family, and how you manage your health, so that you may age well.

To accomplish this however, Americans must first change their overall perception of aging. The process of aging must be understood to represent a privilege and not a burden. The idea that aging allows an opportunity that will not be extended to all comers and that the alternative is really not an option. To eliminate the general misconceptions associated with aging and instead recognize that aging represents a positive phenomenon. In truth the only way to stop the aging process is to die and this is not our goal.

Retailers would have you believe that youth can be purchased in a bottle or that the aging process can be stopped with a pill. The same people who resist their own physicians' legitimate prescriptions are all too eager to try one of these so called remedies. Concoctions, produced in basement laboratories by junior chemists, that carry outrageous claims, are all the rage. These drugs are not regulated, are unproven and cost a bundle. Last year alone over one billion dollars were spent on such products by the American public.

The people who create these products will usually manipulate the truth to accomplish their goals. They may tell us, there are more people alive with heart disease now than ever before and that current medicines have not "cured" heart disease but that their product will correct the problem. They are intentionally manipulating the truth. The truth is, as presented in an earlier chapter of this book, that the population has doubled and now includes a higher percentage of older individuals. This older population also carries the highest incidence of heart disease when compared to other age groups. However, unlike prior generations who succumbed to their heart disease and died because there were no medications available to treat their condition, current generations of elderly persons have been kept alive as a direct result of the medications that are now available to them. Therefore, based on this reality, it would be true to state that there are more people alive with heart disease today than ever before. It is however, inaccurate to manipulate this fact and state that current medications have therefore been ineffective in combating this disease, since there are more cases of disease now then ever before. Or to go one step further and claim that "their so called medication" will therefore work better.

In addition, some retailers will state that modern medicine has not produced a cure for such illnesses as heart disease. This statement would be accurate. There is no cure for heart disease. However, the retailers' insinuation suggests that the medical community has misinformed or failed its patients. I am not aware of any medical organization which has ever made such a claim. Rather, current medications have been created and used successfully to treat the potentially deadly symptoms associated with such diseases, not cure the illness. These medications have thereby allowed such afflicted individuals to live for a longer period of time with a better quality of life. Not bad for nothing more than a bunch of poisons deliberately devised to milk the American public of their money.

The point is that people want a reason to believe that everything is possible. I chose to believe that nothing is impossible. Although most people would say that these statements are the same, they are quite different. The former suggest unbridled or unfounded exuberance and blind faith whereas the latter implies cautious optimism, study and promise. Not the promises served up in a cleverly designed bottle or by some con-artist, but rather the promises provided through facts, studies and science. Promises realized only through time and effort for the betterment of mankind!

The study of aging is only in its infancy and although there is much to learn, the important point is, the process has begun. There will be multiple issues to address and investigate as we move forward. Many of the current theories and concepts regarding aging will have to change for such research to be successful. The necessary adjustments will, I have no doubt, occur. Establishing the appropriate mindset necessary to succeed remains the most challenging proposition. However, once this is realized, the field of medicine will demonstrate miraculous accomplishments through the study of aging within the next ten years.

Research studies have already identified that people with better health before age sixty-five experience decreased disability after age sixty-five. However, relatively little attention has been given to this fact. Perhaps the researchers felt that this represents nothing more than the obvious. In reality however, it identifies the fact that a larger proportion of people are not only reaching the age of sixty-five but arriving under better circumstances with regard to their health. It suggests that a method to accomplish better aging does indeed exist and that we can incorporate such methods, through the use of knowledge, into our lives.

Given the appropriate opportunity, the BHS Factor can produce significant positive changes in your life today and in the future. However, little will be gained from reading this material and not fully grasping the knowledge and power that it offers. The knowledge to limit disability and maintain independence while improving future health and quality of life is, in and of itself, enlightening. The ability to effectively change what has been deemed unchangeable, to reach the unreachable, is empowering.

The desire for extended life has long been an ambition of the human condition. Yet, few people are actually willing to recognize that with every wish there often comes a curse. The "wish" of longevity is being realized today, but the disability, pain, dementia and general loss of independence currently associated with longevity serves as the "curse." These conditions and consequences are not acceptable and must be improved upon in the future. We are not looking for a "cure" but rather an acceptable alterative.

# *Section II*

# CHAPTER 8

▼

# "BACK TO THE FUTURE"

The first section of this book has thus far been dedicated to establishing, in a manner of speaking, "the facts of life". The regurgitation of information aimed at heightening awareness of the possible consequences that may come with aging. A virtual tour through currently available data, predicted future expectations, and an occasional "opinion" or two. An opportunity to identify the potential pitfalls that can be expected with aging, as well as, investigate possible solutions.

The data reviewed thus far has hopefully provided crucial information and insight to the future of aging. It not only indicates that the current population is getting older but that the baby boomer generation will live longer the current aged population. In addition, this data clearly shows the high incidence of disability associated with aging, the negative effect it exerts on individuals and the toll it places on society. On the other hand, it also offers hidden treasure. Although, based on this data, the consequences of aging have been demonstrated to not be reversible there is clear indication that they are preventable.

The potential value of this knowledge is immeasurable. It literally means that we have the power to change the future. Unfortunately, for many of us, this becomes a difficult concept to fully comprehend. In other words, because we have not seen the future, we cannot fully comprehend how we might be able to change its course. We have no point of reference and therefore nothing to measure or compare to.

A great example of this can be seen in the fictional movie *Back to the Future*. In this movie Dr. Emmit Brown creates a time travel machine from a car, namely a Delorian. The main character, Marty Mcfly, then uses this contraption to not only go back in time but to then return back to the future. In the movie, Marty Mcfly, in visiting the past, is able to influence his future. He is allowed the opportunity to experience his home life at the beginning and the end of the movie and witness first hand the positive influence that he had created by visiting and changing his past.

Unfortunately, it is unlikely that we will have access to a time machine to experience exactly how we might influence and change our futures. Let alone a time machine made from a Delorian. How far fetched is that? However, in-spite of not being afforded the luxury of a before and after assessment of the future, we need to realize that our actions influence our futures just the same. This is the power that the BHS Factor will have on our lives.

Therefore, the second section of this book will focus on how to identify and incorporate the BHS Factor into our own lives. In effect, to design a plan that will allow us the opportunity to harness the power of the BHS Factor and take advantage of the potential it can offer our individual futures. Through the implementation of relatively simple lifestyle changes, we can enjoy better health now and activate the long term benefits of the BHS Factor for later. It will actually allow us an opportunity to enjoy our newfound longevity rather than just suffer through it.

The BHS Factor will require the implementation of a host of other factors to produce results. Theses factors represent the story within the story or rather the roots of the BHS Factor. Although they will be discussed separately, in the end it will become quite evident how they manage to influence each other. In fact, it will become quite clear that these factors actually accentuate each other and will therefore produce synergy.

# CHAPTER 9

▼

# THE BHS FACTOR

Section 9.1    *Health Factor*

Section 9.2    *Lifestyle Factor*

Section 9.3    *Behavioral Factor*

Section 9.4    *Mental Factor*

Section 9.5    *Spiritual Factor*

Section 9.6    *Social-Economic Factor*

Section 9.7    *Dimensionality Factor*

# *9.1 HEALTH FACTOR*

As previously discussed most people take their health for granted. Little or no thought is given to the little changes that occur to our bodies through the years. In most cases, people don't think about growing old but rather assume that it is a process that just happens. In-fact, we typically expect this process to occur, but in general, it is to far off in the future to concern ourselves now.

Inevitably, every one of us will, sooner or later, associate a negative physical experience with an expected consequence of aging. The standard, "I must be getting old" is a customarily acceptable excuse in such cases. This attitude however produces complacency and allows us to accept the abnormal as normal. What this means is that we accept minor physical changes as unavoidable conditions of aging and do little or nothing about them. Eventually these minor changes, not having been corrected, come to represent major changes to our persona.

The best examples I can provide of just such situations and the toll they can have on a person occurred to both my father and uncle when I was a teenager. Upon waking up one morning and attempting to raise out of bed, my father experienced lower back pain. Of course, he thought nothing of it and felt that this was just a "minor" back ache. It would seem to make sense; after all, he worked as a cook and was on his feet for ten to twelve hours a day in a hot kitchen.

To my father and most of the working class of his generation, the back ache represented nothing more than a consequence of the job. This learned mentality, coupled with the belief that he just wasn't as young as he used to be, permitted my father to actually do nothing to address his back problem. He did not see a doctor, take time off from work, or even consider using a medication. Instead, he created his own solution for his back problem. He noticed that the pain in his lower back could be reduced or eliminated by simply shifting the position of his upper back. The abnormal was now normal. Soon his posture was completely corkscrewed and cockeyed. It wasn't long before he was having additional muscle-skeletal problems that would lead to further disabilities.

A similar circumstance occurred to my uncle. He woke up one morning and headed for the bathroom where he noticed his urinary flow was slower than usual. He later explained that at the time he remembered, snickering to himself, and thinking that he was getting old. Less than two years later the urinary flow stopped completely. He was rushed to the hospital and found to have an obstruction of his urinary system. In addition, he had developed acute renal failure and hydronephrosis or an enlargement of the kidneys as a result of this blockage or obstruction. The blockage was eventually corrected with relatively minor surgery and the hydronephrosis also resolved as a result. However, his kidney function was only partially corrected. He was therefore required to take medication in order to help maintain his kidney function. Unfortunately, this medication caused several side-effects, in particular, he now found himself incontinent of urine. Due to his embarrassment, as a result of his incontinence, he discontinued the medicine. This in-turn caused his kidney function to decline rapidly and he soon died as a result.

These situations unfortunately occur every morning of everyday and they represent classic examples of our ignorance regarding our own individual health. My father's situation can easily be equated with having a bothersome stone or pebble in his shoe. Instead of removing it, he chose to alter his walking style to avoid the discomfort that the pebble was causing. Who in their right mind would not remove a pebble from their shoe to avoid having to compensate their posturing?

In my uncle's case, a condition which could have easily been corrected instead went neglected until it caused permanent damage. The initial decreased urinary flow that my uncle experienced represented nothing more than the equivalent of having a kink in a garden hose that was slowing the flow of water. The question was simply whether to un-kink the hose or choose to do nothing, he obviously chose incorrectly.

Albert Einstein, once said, "The difference between genius and stupidity is that genius has its limits." Although now long gone, I still
carry the utmost respect for my father and uncle, and consider both of
them as having been intelligent men. However, their respective decisions in these situations were pure and simple examples of stupidity. In
both cases, these conditions occurred before age sixty-five. In both
cases, the causative factors producing the problems were easily treatable
and reversible. In both cases, the results brought about specific compromises and complications after age sixty-five.

How often do we wakeup with similar minor ailments and "walk
them off" or convince ourselves that we're "just getting old." Based on
such attitudes, it should come as no surprise to us on that fateful morning that we wake up and realize that we "feel" old and therefore we are
old. The point is that these physical changes that we will inevitably
experience represent signals. They are the body's method of trying to
tell us that we may need to somehow intervene to break the cycle and
prevent possible progression of a minor condition. We need to pay
attention to what our bodies are telling us.

However, most people choose to determine how they feel based on
their chronological age. In other words, since the invention of the calendar, people have associated age with the number of days they've been
on the planet. In-turn, chronological age has served to define our
expected health status for a given age. In reality one has nothing to do
with the other. On the other hand, biological age is not a reflection of
measure but rather how well our bodies continue to function both
mentally and physically. It serves as a more accurate indicator of our
true health status and how we feel physically. The bodies function is
not a consequence of chronological aging, a person does not automatically fall apart on their fortieth birthday.

Rather, aging is a developmental process based on biological function. In our daily lives, we are all acquainted with someone who is sixty
years of age or older, whether a parent, grand-parent, friend, or associate. Through simple observation, of these folks, we must recognize that

some of them function at the biological age of a forty year old, while others more closely resemble a person much older than their stated age. This contrast of physical conditions in people of the same age represents the essence of biological aging and the potential ability to manipulate the aging process.

Less than two decades ago, athletes were regarded over-the-hill at twenty-five years of age. Today however, they are considered to only be reaching the peak of their performance at age twenty-eight to thirty. For the very same reasons that super-athletes are able to perform better and for longer periods or careers, the average person can realize better longevity. The biological process allows us the ability to rise above our chronological age and the false limitations we have placed on ourselves by using a calendar to measure our age.

Physicians have long viewed the biological processes of the body as the system that dictates how we age and the explanation for why we age so differently. In truth, under "normal" conditions we age quite similarly! In fact, the life span or biological limit of human life is estimated to be 150 years if a person lives free of disease and social interference. It is important to realize that the factor which distinguishes a healthy eighty year old from a decrepit individual of the same age is pathological aging. Pathology, as a result of exposure to disease, social insult, and major stress, remains the basic cause of accelerated aging.

Science and technology have played an immense role in successfully treating and in some cases eliminating such pathology. People today live longer as a direct result of vaccinations, antibiotics, hormones, insulin, and other medical advances. These medical advances represent a large part of the equation. However, to complete the equation it is up to us to actively participate and assume accountability for our individual healthcare.

As I write this, the major news channels on television are reporting a story that serves as a perfect example of exactly what I am stating here. There is an obese woman who has lodged a complaint with the State Medical Board against her doctor. This woman who is, at a minimum, fifty to sixty pounds overweight, claims that the physician advised her that she was to fat and needed to lose weight to improve her overall health. This is the same person who would turn around and file a lawsuit against her doctor if she were to have a massive heart attack, claiming she was not appropriately advised to lose weight during routine physicals. This is a person who is in denial and lacks balance in her life. The point is quite simply that science and technology have brought the information to the table, now it is up to us to use this information to help ourselves.

Future generations will be required to actively participate directly in their healthcare. We should not be surprised if the day comes when, just like life insurance, you may not qualify for medical insurance because of your weight, cigarette smoking, nonparticipation in a routine exercise program, etc. Some insurance companies may actually not cover an illness if you are not proactively participating in an established preventative health program.

Active participation in preventative health practices can aid in the avoidance of pathological aging and the pitfalls which may compromise health and longevity. Routine medical examinations, including physicals, laboratory studies, chest X-rays and electrocardiograms, are essential. Early diagnosis and intervention of minor health issues can prevent major life altering events which can cut our lives short.

One of the greatest assets afforded to us as Americans is our availability to information. The field of medicine has identified "best practices" which can be used to monitor and preserve our health. This data offers the best possible outcomes for the population when specific medical and non-medical health interventions are appropriately implemented. A person's conscious decision to not take advantage of this knowledge and expertise is nothing short of ludicrous.

## *Health Factor Rules*

**-Take responsibility for your health.**

   -Accept Accountability!
   -Make your own decisions based on facts.
   -Second opinions are your Right.

**-Do not accept abnormal as normal.**

   -There are no unavoidable conditions of aging.
   -Don't trivialize "minor" aliments.

**-Minor ailments require your attention.**

   -Treat illness when it occurs. Don't Wait!
   -Most minor aliments are reversible early.

**-Listen to what your body is telling you.**

   -Preserve your body's function.
   -Avoid Over-Stress. Make time for yourself.
   -Avoid Social Insult (drugs-pollution-tobacco)

**-Invest in Preventative Medicine.**

   -Establish routine medical visits.
   -Adhere to routine medical screening tests.

**-Alternative Medicine is Supplemental.**

   -Nontraditional forms of medicine should
   **NOT** be considered acceptable first line treatment choices.
   -Alternative medicine should only be used as
   an adjunct to traditional medicine and only
   when proven to *cause no harm*.

## BHF Factor Recommendations *for* Routine Medical Care

If your Forty years old and have not had a routine physical exam, you need to have one done now! Here is a list of what you should have included as part of your routine physical.

| | |
|---|---|
| Breast Exam | Yearly |
| Mammogram | |
| Rectal Exam | Yearly |
| Occult Blood | |
| PAP Smears | Yearly |

Laboratory Tests
   **Cholesterol**
   **Liver function**
   **Complete Blood Count**
   **Kidney Function**
   **Electrolytes**
   **Thyroid Studies**
Chest X-ray
EKG
Hearing Test
Vision Test
**Yearly Medical Physical Exams are recommended after the age 45.**

## 9.2 LIFESTYLE FACTOR

Obviously the medical profession has realized the importance of lifestyle changes on the human condition. However, over the years, the encouraged evolution of lifestyle changes upon our population has appeared to be nothing less than tragic. Physicians and all other healthcare professionals have touted diet and exercise in one form or another to promote health. The results of this quest, to say the least, have not been impressive. Recent statistics suggest that we are the fattest nation in the world and that 50 percent of the population, including kids, is obese.[13] We also carry the distinction of being the most sedentary nation as well. In addition, in-spite of fast food restaurants efforts to take over the planet and corrupt other civilizations, we still have the highest fat contents in our diets. The inevitable markings of a modern day society.

Through the years, the type of exercise recommended by health professionals has been quite varied. This is predominantly a result of physicians overall ignorance regarding this area. It was not so long ago that extreme exercise programs were being touted as the answer to our obesity. The inability of most persons to adhere to such programs and the relative damage caused as a result of such excess soon had physicians recommending moderate exercise as the new found answer to our dilemma. Now the recommendation is to walk. Yes, walk your excess pounds away or walk your way to health. Can such a low maintenance program help accomplish such lofty goals?

The answer surprisingly enough is yes. Walking can produce significant positive results to a person's overall health status. In the past, most people could not endure the more strenuous programs recommended by their physicians. In fact, they should consider themselves lucky if they were sensible enough to have settled for abstinence. On the other hand, if they weren't so lucky, they found themselves suffering with potentially significant injuries from over stressed joints and other musculoskeletal injuries. The fact is that the populations of most other countries maintain their weight, stamina and endurance simply because they walk. They have not become inherently dependent on modern conveniences as we have in this country. For example, most Europeans may own a vehicle but many will rarely use them. They electively choose to walk, they don't really even think about it, it's a mind set. The reasons why Europeans actually walk maybe several fold. However, whether by preference or necessity, such as the high cost of gas, the end result is overall better health.

A recent newspaper article reported what was described as a "significant discovery" for our times. Small populations of people who live in a remote mountainous village were found to have prolonged life expectancies with less disability. The article went on to say that scientists were anxious to study the people of this village and identify their secret to longevity. The answer is quite simply that they do not suffer the consequences of "industrial disease." They have no other form of transportation except their legs, they consume low fat diets and eat primarily off the land, their air is clean, and their water pure. Try walking a mountain twice a day, to pick food and haul water, and see if you're not healthier within four weeks. You might be astonished how such simplicity might actually advance your life.

Diets on the other hand have become anything but simple. Low fat, no carbohydrates, Mediterranean diets, South Beach diets, cards, points, you name it and someone has tried it. The true solution, is plain old school know how. Stop over eating and sitting on your ass! The amounts of food that we throw in the trash each year could feed several nations. The excess calories we consume on a daily bases represent upwards of 10 pounds of additional weight we will gain per year. It is impossible that we as a nation can be this hungry all the time.

The bottom line is simply to eat less. I have struggled with weight my whole life and have only found eating less to produce results. A low fat, reduced carbohydrate diet works just fine if you stay in the range of 1200 calories per day. Once you have reached your weight loss goals increase your intake to 2200 calories or so depending on your level of activity and this will keep you at your desired weight. Obviously, this old school philosophy of eat less and do more must work, considering that prior generations did not carry the distinction of being labeled the fattest population on the planet. In addition, avoid foods with saturated and trans fats, reduce carbohydrates, and avoid "white foods" such as white flour, sugar and salt. These items should be eliminated or significantly reduced from your diet.

Possibly of even greater importance to our diets and general overall health is what we tend to drink. Beverages which contain carbonation and artificial sweeteners represent the worst possible ingredients we can place in our bodies. These ingredients have been shown to actually attack our joints, deplete the body of essential minerals, and promote weight gain. Americans however feel an overwhelming need to keep the major soda companies in business and drink billions of gallons of this crap per year. Plain and simple, it's not good for you! Your body doesn't need flavor, sugar, artificial sweetener, or carbonation, it only needs water. Drink eight ounces of distilled water eight times per day. Before you ponder the question, yes coffee and tea, preferably green tea consumption, in moderation, are ok.

The harsh reality is that few of us will adhere to a strict diet all the time. It probably also goes without saying that most of us will never realize our ideal body weight. These unfortunate realizations however should not serve as our excuse to not eat a proper diet. For most of us, simply reducing the amount of food we currently eat will probably result in immediate beneficial weight loss. The benefits from simply exchanging what we are currently drinking for distilled water are immeasurable. If such diet modifications are implemented in conjunction with increased activity, such as walking for 20 minutes two times per day, you will have improved your overall health for the future.

Life style changes don't have to be dramatic to produce results. The answer lies in just getting started and sticking with it. Being 10 pounds over weight and active will always carry a health advantage over the person who is 20 pounds overweight and sedentary. Once you realize results and feel generally better or healthier, I am confident that you're new found logical thinking will instruct you to take the next steps. Not only to improve the quality of food you eat but to further reduce the quantity consumed.

In addition, you will feel so good about yourself that you will find alternate methods to increase your activity levels and actually enjoy doing it. Your goals will no longer seem unattainable or unreachable but rather you will be accomplishing realistic goals you have set for yourself. Most of us realize that exercise carried out as repetitive movements can quickly become a monotonous chore. Therefore, the idea is to think in terms of continuous motion. Go for a walk, mow the lawn, rake the leaves, stand instead of sit, sit instead of lying down, jog, play catch with the kids, clean the garage, the list of things you can do is endless. Coming home from work and feeling a need to relax or unwind is common and natural. Now, instead of sitting in front of the television, or having a cocktail to unwind, get in motion! Eliminate old habits and incorporate new ones. You will find that continues motion is more invigorating and that at the conclusion of the activity you will actually feel more relaxed and energetic.

The benefits of exercise cannot be stressed enough. Exercise will counteract the supposed inevitable effects of aging and improve quality of life. Increased motion during our forties and fifties is the key to better health after sixty-five. The reason that increased motion can have such a profound effect on our lives now and in the future is multi-factorial. However, the two most significant reasons are, this routine will help in establishing a positive behavior that will continue throughout the remainder of our lives and the fact that motion preserves flexibility. It is loss of flexibility which, by and large, hinders our ability to carry-out activities of daily living. Preserving flexibility is of utmost importance to achieving our goal of limiting future disability and thereby aging successfully.

## *Lifestyle Factor Rules*

### -Take responsibility for your health.

-Make your own decisions based on facts.
-Stop saying you can't, you know you can.
-Commit to improving yourself.

### -Get up and do something!

-Motion is crucial to maintaining flexibility.
-Flexibility is crucial to maintaining function.
-Exercise should not be a chore.
-Chores can serve as exercise.
-Think European, park the car and walk.

### -Improve your diet.

-Learn how to decipher food labels.
-Eliminate fats. (Saturated and Trans fats)
-Reduce carbohydrates.
-Eliminate White foods.
-Eliminate drinks with carbonation.
-Eliminate drinks with artificial sweeteners.
-Invest in a commercial weight loss program.

### -Listen to what your body is telling you.

-Cut down on calories. Stop overeating!
-Buy distilled water and actually drink it!
-If you believe it, your body will follow.

# 9.3 BEHAVIORAL FACTOR

The ability to change our behaviors will potentially present the greatest challenge. The reason for this is simply that behaviors are usually nothing more than habits or rituals that we repeat over and over again. They represent what we have chosen to incorporate into our daily lives and have become accepted as routine. Behavior represents the ultimate act of doing without thinking and therefore it is difficult for many people to deviate from the routine which has become imbedded in their minds and which now represents the established norm.

Our lives are filled with repetitive cycles that are carried out over and over again without actually having to think through the process. If we were required to repeatedly think our way through these daily cycles it would be exacerbating. As a safety mechanism the brain defers such routine activities and by doing so they thereby become unconscious tasks. Thankfully the mind realizes that repeatedly thinking through the mundane will make you insane.

Learned behaviors are as implied, learned over time and implanted into our brains until they are basically automatic. Although this process is different from basic primal functioning of the brain which is used for a number of bodily functions, such as breathing, it will help to establish the difficulty that maybe encountered when trying to change a routine behavior. For example, as indicated, breathing is a primal function carried out by the brain. The cycle is simple, breath in and breath out, our bodies or more specifically our lungs repeat this cycle on average of 20 times per minute, 1200 times per hour, or over 28,000 times per day. It occurs automatically and therefore is an unconscious exercise that requires no thinking. However, if you were to try and consciously monitor your breathing and reduce the rate down to 10 cycles per minute, even for a short two minute interval, you might find the experience frustrating and quite frankly exhausting. The same holds true when trying to change a learned behavior, it will require effort.

Learned behaviors are evident in just about everything we do and actually play a part in what, when, and how we carryout tasks. The old adage, "it's hard to teach an old dog new tricks" obviously holds true. Learning new behaviors will require thought and repetitiveness to eventually become routine. The simplest task can suddenly become stressful or even difficult to complete when we are forced to break from the usual accepted mode of operation. The classic example of this type phenomenon is seen in the workplace while observing new hires trying to adapt to an unfamiliar environment. The large sums of money expended by major companies to train new employees and the high rate of trainees who are unable to cope or comply with such training is case and point.

Learned behaviors simply become part of a routine and are therefore difficult to change. This holds true regardless of whether such unconscious behaviors are positive or negative influences in our lives. Therefore, if we are to realize our goals it will become necessary for us to incorporate the basic principle and belief that the mode and method of completing any task can be improved upon. Even the simplest tasks have established methods that have been found to be more effective when implemented. For example, the American Dental Association has a specific protocol for brushing teeth and yet although many of us brush our teeth, few of us follow the recommended proven procedure. The general acceptance that minimal changes, such as brushing up and down rather than side to side and brushing three times a day rather than once a day or brushing once a day rather than not at all, can produce positive results in our daily routines must be understood. I chose dental hygiene, to over emphasize the point! However, the truth is quite simply that there is always room for improvement regardless of the action or task being carried out. In fact, there is most likely a better way of completing any task whether it is considered simple and routine or complex and unusual.

On a completely different level, another example of a learned behavior is cigarette smoking. Although it's true that cigarettes are addictive, the reality is that we are not born ready to smoke. Rather, this activity is introduced as a behavior into our lives and in doing so an addiction is formed. Yet, smokers don't usually light up a cigarette because they are craving nicotine. Rather, smokers light up as a result of social unconsciousness. In other words, social events induce the use, morning coffee…morning cigarette; driving in the car…light up a cigarette; have a beer…have a cigarette. This unconscious activity represents the habit as a behavior. The behavior only serves to reinforce the habit as an addiction. This process holds true for many activities, including alcohol consumption, eating, television, etc.

Obviously, the consequences associated with smoking are real and the health benefits associated with smoke cessation cannot be overstated. However, although the best option is to quit, most smokers have heard this before and have not followed such advice. Therefore, would it not make sense that tobacco reduction might prove just as beneficial in such situations? The implication, simply being, reduced participation, with regard to a "bad" habit, might also hold potential benefit. It would only seem logical that decreased cigarette intake from one pack per day to half a pack per day would be of greater benefit than not doing anything at all. Obviously, bad habits should be broken and thereby eliminated from our lives. However, any intervention can serve as a stepping stone towards accomplishing a long range goal. For example, if a smoker were to reduce their consumption by 3 cigarettes per day this would represent approximately 1100 less cigarettes or 55 packs in the first year alone. Who would say this is not an improvement? The introduction of any program dedicated to the reduced participation in such negative habits should be viewed as a positive. Regardless of whether they are carried out gradually over time or achieved cold turkey.

Such accomplishments represent positive influences to our overall well being. However, they are not easily attained or, for that matter, sustained even when they come to represent the new routine. There has to be an accepted underlying belief that such changes are not only positive but come with an associated long term benefit. For many people this means additional motivation or incentive will be required to accomplish such goals. As a physician, I unconsciously wash my hands after visiting each patient. This routine not only provides a benefit to my patients but also serves to prevent me from contracting potential illnesses. Therefore, aside from the responsibility to my patients, there is an additional incentive to wash my hands in that it will protect me as well.

For this same reason, I am always a little unsettled when walking into the restroom of my favorite restaurant. There, on the mirror above the sink, a sign has been posted to alert the employees that they must wash their hands before returning to work. The truth is, if a person does not usually wash their hands after using the toilet for their own protection, the expectation that they will routinely do so as an employee because of a posted sign is nothing more than wishful thinking. There is no added incentive to the individual to carryout this task, and therefore no motivation to follow this command. Incentives provide the motivation we need to succeed.

It is also essential to understand that after introducing a new task to our daily schedule it must eventually become second nature or, in other words, routine for this process to prove successful. For example, if we decide to eliminate saturated fats from our diet, there must come a point where we no longer have to think about our actions for the task to be successfully accomplished. The same holds true for exercise. For instance, if we initiate a walking or jogging program, the first week might be filled with enthusiasm. However, rest assured, the second week will be filled with aches, pains, and dread. By the third week, or the "week of procrastination," many of us will be searching for any possible excuse to avoid having to exercise. Hopefully, however, by the forth week we should realize we can accomplish this task and that we can actually block out of our minds any potential negative thoughts that would deter us from doing so. By week five it should become routine, in much the same manner that we would wake up and make coffee, brush our teeth or comb our hair. At this point the task has become a normal daily practice.

The conclusion therefore is basically simple. Whether adding a positive or eliminating a negative the method remains the same. The mechanism of thought or having to rethink the process must eventually be eliminated to achieve success. Only when the desired behavior becomes second nature or routine can it thereby become established in our lives and produce a positive influence in our existence.

## *Behavioral Factor Rules*

### -Changing behaviors require effort.

-Change requires thought and repetition.
-Repetition eventually becomes routine.
-Any task can be improved upon.

### -Incentives provide motivation!

-Motivation + Incentive = Success.
-Exercise and reward yourself.
-Eat right and reward yourself.
-Help yourself find your inner potential.

### -Eliminate Negatives!

-Reduction is better than no change at all.
-Everything in moderation is acceptable.
-Stop smoking! Ask for help if you need it!

# *9.4 MENTAL FACTOR*

In-spite of evidence to the contrary, as indicated by the evermore bizarre Newspaper Headlines and apparent craziness of the world, mans greatest asset is his ability to think. The human brain is always at work both consciously and subconsciously. For the most part it does a relatively good job of guiding us through our day. The brain controls every function of our body, from hormones and thinking, to body movement, senses and emotions. As a result, there is also an ever present opportunity for things to go wrong.

The human brain is not a cloned entity but rather it controls us in as much as we control it. What this suggests is that apart from the brain growing physically, the brain's ability to function is a developed quality. This evolution relies not only on information we provide the brain through education, but is also a function of the society in which we live and our life experiences. The brain interprets this information and develops conclusions which in-turn determines how we envision, react and fit into the world. In a manner of speaking, the brain through its interpretation of such information eventually develops into a mind. Therefore, while the brain represents a purely physical object, the mind suggests a process. Ultimately the mind determines who we are as individuals.

While the human mind is obviously a wondrous accomplishment, it is quite liable. Whether this is a consequence of the brains physical fragility or the stresses of the outside world or both is unknown for certain. The fact is that our reaction to any situation will be variable and completely dependent on the affects of stressors on our minds or the malfunctioning circuitry of our brains. A person can become enraged over an incident that produced laughter a week before or emotional for no apparent reason and unable to explain why they are crying or upset. Simply put the mind can and will mess with you.

Mental fluctuations, such as emotional outbursts, produce instability that directly affects our behaviors. Eventually such situations lead to the development of more serious mental conditions. These types of conditions present themselves throughout a person's life and are recognizable in varying forms. For example, a young person who develops Anorexia Nervosa and an older person who becomes severely depressed are possibly influenced by the minds same distortional perceptions. In other words, the minds inability to cope with a specific situation or stressor produces an alternate condition to divert its attention from the primary issue. These types of secondary reactions occur all the time but in many instances go unnoticed. It is important that we occasionally take a moment to step back and examine the what, where, why and how of our thinking.

If one accepts the theory that the human mind is a process and dependent on the brain to function, it becomes evident that the mind is indeed quite fragile. The mind is only as good as the brains circuitry allows it to be. Therefore, the horsepower that the brain provides us can be quite a variable entity and the principle reason why people function as they do. The explanation as to why some people can cope with the most extreme of circumstances while others struggle with the simplest of tasks. The mind is therefore dependent on conservation of the brain.

Based on this assumption, it should become readily apparent that in order to maintain brain function we must preserve brain matter. Unfortunately, the human brain has been shown to shrink in size as we age. Although, there are many postulated theories regarding this phenomena, it would appear that the "don't use it and lose it" theory describes it best. The theory simply states that as we age we tend not to use our minds as often or as aggressively as we do during middle age and therefore the brain shrinks. This shrinkage in-turn is believed to produce progressive deterioration of thought and memory. Based on such a presumption, it would thereby appear that preserving brain matter is codependent on maintaining brain function.

Preservation of mental health is and will be essential to our future wellbeing. Cognitive impairment or dementia currently affects approximately 4.5 million individuals in the United States.[14] Dementia is a primary reason for loss of independence and the associated prolonged morbidity. Cognitive impairment represents a major enemy in our fight towards aging with dignity. Arriving into our elder years physically intact but not being able to think will not serve us well. As a physician, I witness first hand the devastating consequences such scenarios' pose on both patients and families everyday. We as individuals, as well as, our immediate family must become educated so that we can identify and intervene when the mind is possibly malfunctioning.

Forgetfulness, wondering, altered thinking and bizarre behaviors warrant immediate investigation by a physician. Simple screening tests exist to evaluate patients for dementia and they should be included as part of your routine yearly physical examination. Early recognition and treatment have proven extremely beneficial in delaying disease progression. Contrary to popular beliefs, many people are able to identify changes associated with dementia relatively early on in the process. The reality however is that few people do anything to intervene until after they are subjected to a crisis as a result of their advancing disease. This is a trend that must be reversed and permanently ended for there to be success in our pursuit of quality of life in our old age.

It is also important to realize that there are other mental illnesses that can occur among the elderly population besides dementia. Mood disorders, anxiety, psychosis and depression often go undiagnosed and untreated. These conditions can limit physical, mental and social functioning and interfere with normal day to day performance. In-turn these potentially treatable illnesses can represent the beginning of the end for many aged individuals. Consider this; approximately fifteen percent of the elderly population suffers with these conditions and this has been calculated to be equivalent to slightly more than all cancer patients for all ages. It is therefore imperative that we learn to identify these mental illnesses, as well as, eliminate the concerns related to social stigmas associated with these conditions. Mental illness must be treated as early in the process as possible and should be treated aggressively. As with dementia, the rule is simply, the earlier the prescribed intervention the better the potential outcome. Neglecting to recognize these disorders allows for pronounced and prolonged morbidity, not mortality. This basically means an opportunity to live a long life with disability while only wishing we were dead. The purpose of the BHS Factor is to avoid just this scenario.

# *Mental Factor Rules*

## -Take responsibility for your health.

-Make your own decisions based on facts.
-Educate yourself about mental illnesses.
-Make your doctor screen for dementia yearly.

## -The mind relies on the brain!

-Limit alcohol consumption.
-Don't use recreational drugs ever!
-Avoid head injuries. (Seat belts, helmets.)

## -Use it or lose it!

-Stimulate your brain by reading, math, etc.

## -Your brain works better when you...

-Reduce stress,
-Exercise,
-Eat right.
-Meditate, learn to enjoy silence.

## -Listen to what your body is telling you.

-Early detection is key to treating mental ills.
-If you notice changes seek professional help.
-Pay attention to the little things.
-Nothing is trivial.
-Don't take anything for granted.

# 9.5 SPIRITUAL FACTOR

The following section involves discussion that addresses what I will refer to as spiritual factors. This topic can present many emotions and ideals for many people. Therefore, for the purpose of our discussion spiritual factors will represent those "things" which provide us inner peace. But, what exactly is inner peace? Words such as tranquility, serenity and harmony have all been used to define peace. If such words serve as true representatives, then peace is, without question, the true underlying essence of life.

The intrinsic similarities or the outward diversity of a society and its people define what inner peace or harmony might represent to the individual members of such a community. These variables stem from different backgrounds, religious beliefs, traditions and so on. In some circles however these differences are often looked upon as a hindrance, rather than being recognized for the true wonders of living which they represent.

Over the course of our lives most of us will experience multiple events, both positive and negative, that will influence the direction we travel during the journey of life. However, how such events touch and eventually affect us will ultimately depend on our inner peace. This inner peace therefore will dictate and direct our perceptions, interpretation and reactions to everything we experience during our lifetimes.

Whether an event enriches our lives or depletes and drains us, depends on our self-confidence and underlying self-esteem. People with low self-esteem are usually negative by nature; they lack self-confidence and therefore have a distorted perception of themselves and the world that surrounds them. Such perceptions in-turn will skew their views and interpretation of events and thereby only allow for negative interactions or reactions. These people are, in one form or another, generally insatiable, preoccupied, self-absorbed, or overall angry individuals. These are the people that I refer to as, the "lost souls of society". Regardless of social status, religion, family, etc., these people are convinced that "something" is missing in their lives. They, therefore, are constantly searching for "something" and quite simply that "something" is their inner peace. Unfortunately, in most cases they won't find it until it's too late.

On the other hand, the person with high self-esteem and self-confidence is usually positive by nature. Generally speaking, these people are happy, well adapted, outgoing individuals who love life and the world in which they live. Such persons are not passive or complacent and they are not naive to the problems of the world. Rather, they have found what the others are so desperately searching for. Their inner peace allows them to be optimistic, hopeful, and resilient to events within the world around them, while, more importantly, allowing them the opportunity to comprehend their role within this world.

Only through such realizations can we as individuals, and as a society, improve or possess the desire to improve upon our current status. This desire is crucial to the realization and acceptance of the fact that we were all put on this earth for the betterment of our fellow man. This statement should not be interpreted to represent the beliefs of myself as an individual, a religion or a nation, but rather Humanity. Everything we do will in-turn affect someone else and this process is repeated indefinitely. Some of us may realize wealth while others are subjected to poverty. Some of us may become famous while others live in relative obscurity. These created "conditions" are however insignificant, it is the influence of our inner being on the world that matters.

People repeatedly fail to recognize the significance of their individual influence on the world around them. They tend to trivialize daily activities and marvel only at greatness. When the truth is that through history any person associated with greatness did not just arrive there in place. Rather, these people were molded from birth and undoubtedly influenced by everyone they encountered, and thus developed into what was considered great. I am relatively sure that well known people, who are considered to have made great contributions to humanity, such as George Washington, Martin Luther King, and Thomas Edison met thousands upon thousands of people during their life time. I am also quite confident that the people they encountered before becoming famous represent the influence in their lives that created their greatness and in-turn allowed them the opportunity to touch so many more people. The point is simply that we are all part of a greater horizon.

If at this point you're asking yourself, "what does all this have to do with my health or the BHS factor?" Simply understand that you can either go through life believing that you are being controlled by your environment or that you are, in fact, controlling your environment. Once the basic belief that you have meaning and are contributing to life is understood and accepted, it will become apparent that you are in control of your environment and that you will have achieved the Spirituality Factor. The realization of inner strength, pride, hope and nobility produce inner peace. These qualities, in a manner of speaking, allow us the opportunity to become comfortable within our own skin. They in-turn allow us to realize the inner peace which will guide us through life. In fact, only through the utilization of these virtues can you accomplish that which you desire, successfully.

# *Spiritual Factor Rules*

## -Take responsibility for yourself.

-Make a commitment to improve yourself.
-Realize we have an effect on everything.
-Realize everything around us also affects us.
-Nothing is impossible.
-Anything can happen.
-We can make it happen!

## -Find your Inner Peace!

-Spirituality provides meaning.
-Meaning provides control.
-Control allows contribution to greater cause.
-Self-confidence produces self-esteem.
-Self-esteem produces resilience.
-Don't burn out or fade away, find Balance.

## -Improve yourself!

-Stimulate your brain.
-Reduce stress.
-Exercise.
-Meditate, make time to enjoy silence.
-Eat right.
-Learning behavior requires repetition.

## -Listen to what your body is telling you.

-Frustration produces stress.
-Stress produces anger and negativity.
-Break the cycle before it breaks you.

## 9.6 SOCIAL-ECONOMIC FACTOR

Some of life's realities are not always fair. In this country, more so than others, we are taught at an early age that money makes the world go round. It can be very expensive to live in the "Land of the Free." For many Americans this realization has lead to the creation of the two income household. However, over time two income families have developed into three income families, with a member of the household taking on two or more jobs. Yet, this still is not sufficient for many and eventually these families became more and more dependent on credit. This scenario is an example of a distinctly Capitalist American idea and quite frankly not a "consequence" of other countries. What this has in-turn produced is a society that lives to work as opposed to working to live.

The simple truth is that, except for the ultra-rich, few people are satisfied when it comes to their financial matters. The words from a Bruce Springsteen song states this best, "poor men want to be rich, rich men want to be king and the king's not satisfied until he rules everything". A sad commentary of the human condition, developed as a result of our love of money.

Money or the lack there of, along with education, is what eventually determines our social-economic status. The good news is that both social and economic statuses are not fixed entities. In this country, there is always the opportunity to climb the ladder and achieve financial success. However, it is interesting to note that the proverbial ladder apparently has more than financial benefits according to current economic data. This informational data clearly indicates that health actually improves with increased social and economic status.[15] In other words, the richer you are the healthier you should be.

The indication presented by such reports implies multiple possibilities. The affluent, potentially have better access to healthcare, better knowledge regarding their health, safer home and work environments, improved diets, decreased exposure to toxins and pollutants. All these factors may play a role in improved overall health, but you do not necessarily have to be rich to have such things. Of greater importance is a person's ability to be observant and take advantage of that which is available to them within their own surroundings. This means so much more than utilizing the neighborhood clinic or signing up for local community services. Rather, people need to practice self preservation at every level. Although bringing about such changes may seem difficult, it simply represents a person's underlying perspectives and priorities.

For instance, home safety should be a top priority for all of us. If home is where the heart is and our house is home, then as the commercial says, "We must protect this house." Yet, few of us will invest the time to accomplish this endeavor. For instance, smoke detectors are required through local Building Code Enforcement Agencies. It is common knowledge that these devices should be checked for batteries and overall function on a regular base. This procedure is simple, inexpensive, and can potentially mean the difference between life and death. When was the last time you checked yours? Chances are it has been awhile.

There are literally hundreds of thing that should be evaluated regularly within our homes to ensure our safety. Yet, few people actually safety proof their homes. Every year, millions of Americans are accidentally killed or severely injured in their homes. These are the very same homes that are meant to serve us as shelter. The majority of these accidents are preventable. Instead however, we choose to place ourselves in harms way, because simple routine evaluations of our homes or living space are not carried out on a regular bases. Such inspections have little or nothing to do with money or social status and can prevent the occurrence of catastrophic accidents.

Prevention should serve as our first line of defense in all we do. Whether the topic of discussion is health, safety, finances, etc., prevention through logic should prevail in all these situations. Money has little to do with taking such general precautions. Remember: there is always a better way to accomplish any given task, to avoid an accident, and to prevent a potentially life altering injury. There is real truth in the statement that "an ounce of prevention is worth a pound of cure." Therefore, to realize our goals, we must prioritize our lives and accept accountability for our actions.

As a resident physician in training, I spent a good amount of my time in the emergency ward. On one occasion, I was asked to see a five year old child with a cough who had been brought to the emergency room by his father. The father told me that the cough had been lingering for several weeks and that now it was a cause of concern. After asking several questions of the patient's father, I examined the child but could not find any physical causes for his cough. In addition, during the forty-five minutes spent interviewing the father and examining the child, there was not one single utterance of a cough.

When I asked the father if he had considered taking the child to the hospital clinic during the past several weeks, he said no. When I asked if he had attempted to give the child any over-the-counter medications, such as cough syrup, he again replied no. Now however, he also felt compelled to explain to me how he was working two jobs to make ends meet, that he could not afford the clinic or the cough medicine, and of course that I, as a "rich" physician, could not possibly understand his life and its circumstances. Obviously, he expressed all this in his own special way.

Once he had completed his tirade however, I felt it was my turn to set the record straight and inform him of the actually facts at hand. The truth was that the clinic was Free and available to everyone in the community. In addition, the child's father knew this because, according to the hospital's computer records, the child had been to the clinic in the past for other illnesses and vaccinations. Secondly, I withdrew the pack of cigarettes from his front shirt pocket and suggested in the future he could purchase cough medicine instead. Or, better yet, not purchase cigarettes or learn to smoke them outside his home and that his child would not suffer the consequences of such exposure, namely the cough. I did not feel compelled to explain my origins or my family's plight but I am self assured that I would have won that argument as well.

The moral of the story is simple. People do not always take advantage of the opportunities that are, in many cases, readily available to them. More importantly, and even harder to comprehend, are the people who actually place themselves or their family in harms way by creating potential risk. It doesn't cost a dime to do the right thing.

Although it may be expensive to live in the "Land of the Free", it has more than its share of privileges. In-spite of all its faults, we are free, not only to think for ourselves, but to actually make our own choices. What is merely a dream in many other parts of the world, here in the United States, represents an opportunity to prioritize and influence the significance of our existence. Our lives should be based on basic principles, basic ideas, and doing the right thing. It's not all about the money.

## *Social-Economic Factor Rules*

### -Take responsibility for your life.

-Make your own decisions based on facts.
-Few people are satisfied financially.
-Protect yourself and your family.
-Safeguard your house.
-Safeguard whatever & whenever you can.

### -Life is not always fair!

-Expect the unexpected.
-Don't let finances rule and ruin your life.
-Work to live, don't live to work.

### -Think!

-Practice Safety at home, work and school.
-Reduce risky behavior.
-Plan ahead when you can!

# 9.7 DIMENSIONALITY FACTOR

In this last section the term Dimensionality is used to describe our total lives as human-beings. In essence, the multi-dimensional forces which are continuously at work within us, the positive, negative, good, bad and indifferent. These basic forces that reside within us that influence and thereby promote the development of our perceptions. Perceptions which, in-turn, lead to our ability to survive and adapt to the world in which we live.

Psychologists, psychiatrists, theologians, philosophers, novelists, and poets have written extensively on this very subject. They have used multiple terms to identify and describe this very "essence of man," terms such as self-love, ego, superego, inner-consciousness and soul have been used, just to name a few. In my opinion however, these terms are self-limiting and only represent a small portion of what is described by dimensionality.

In many ways such terms describe a constant or established condition which is unchangeable, an underlying inference that the past not only influences but controls or somehow determines the present. On the other hand, although the concept of dimensionality accepts such wisdom, it also incorporates and expresses the belief that the present as well as the future will significantly influence our past. This simply means that although our current beliefs and perceptions may be based on our past experiences and perceptions, we are also very much influenced by the here and now.

Dimensionality therefore, in a manor of speaking, offers correction for imperfection. For example, the son who blames his cruel mother for his inability to love another woman, or the daughter who adores her father and thereby feels another male cannot replace him in her life, or the obese adolescent who used food as a method to feel better as a child who now continues such practices through their adulthood. Examples such as these are all correctable imperfections. They represent oversimplifications of situations developed by an inferior logic in the immature mind of an adolescent. These situations can all be easily changed or corrected by investigating our past so we may produce and incorporate our futures. The very same reason we study history; to avoid making the same mistakes of the past in the future.

Although for many of you this may appear obvious and straight foreword, it is not that simple. The unconscious mind plays a preeminent role in this process and in many cases people tend to react without thinking. Go to any sixth or seventh grade sporting event and observe the parents watching their children, listen to the comments, body posturing, etc. At the very least, you will walk away amused at the frustration and level of intensity these parents display for what amounts to a meaningless event. Later in your life, or if you have already been in such a situation of parent spectator, examine yourself. You might be surprised to find that your childhood frustrations are suddenly being relived. Only once you think about it will you realize that it exists and only then can you proceed to change it.

The truth is that every seven years or so we, as humans, change both physically and intellectually. Obviously, not all of us grow at the same pace or to a specific required capacity. Physical differences are easily identified by simply observing the different individual body types of everyone around us. Many people can easily identify with that which they can see and they will intervene to compensate for such shortcomings. Mentally the same holds true, some of us will move harmoniously from one level of mental functioning to another without difficulty while others will simply get "stuck." Since these mental differences are more difficult to identify, and the fact that we are not taught or expected to evaluate or reevaluate ourselves through these mental milestones, many of those who get stuck during these periods remain entrenched at these remedial levels. For example, the person who becomes mad, frustrated and argumentative when things are not exactly the way they expect them to be. Such a person has failed to out grow the tantrum phase of a four year old child. This is not to say that they have the mentality of a four year old, but rather that this is a segment of mental growth they did not manage to overcome. The adult mind needs only to identify such behaviors in order to correct them and rise above their adverse effects.

We all have an underlying mental growth milestone that we did not manage to get quite right during our childhood. Yes, that is correct, I said all of us. However, the interference that such handicaps can present in our daily lives is quite variable. Such limitations can present as insignificant events or potentially produce life altering consequences. Unfortunately, many people do not recognize these mental compromises and live their lives in denial, accepting the unacceptable. As an exercise, next time everyone, whether at home or at work, perceives that there is a problem, try to explain why you can't seem to see it. Are they all wrong? Or is it that you might be wrong? Don't waste your time thinking too much about it, the answer is obviously simple.

There is little doubt that our past life experiences affect our day to day behavior. Thankfully, more often than not, the results are positive. However, when past influences affect our lives in negative ways, we must be able to identify them so that we can correct them. We as individuals need to evaluate and re-evaluate ourselves constantly. We are not stationary or static beings, we are constantly being challenged and conflicted by the world we live in. Therefore, taking time to examine our lives is crucial to our existence. There are questions we need to ask and answers we need to know. Why am I angry? Why are we always fighting? Why am I constantly eating? Why do I smoke? Why can't I keep a job? Why am I afraid? Why can't I sleep? Why can't I relax? There are answers to each and every one of these questions. They only need to be logically investigated. We must learn to challenge ourselves to identify these problems so we can seek appropriate solutions. Such problems will not simply go away.

So why is this important to the BHS Factor? Simply put, dimensionality allows us to, not only, better understand our past and how it affects us today. It also allows us the ability to retrain our brain so we can be more productive and better people to ourselves and others. It allows us an opportunity to love ourselves, stroke our ego's, deal with our conscious, and enlighten our souls. It allows an opportunity to be the best we can be. This will not only be reflected upon others but also influence our own directives in a positive manner. Dimensionality allows us to place proper perspective on what is of value and of importance within our lives. I have literally seen such enlightenment change how people interpret everything in the world around them. These people are now able to celebrate life as apposed to just dealing with it. For these people, dimensionality has reduced the stress that comes with or is associated with "just" living.

Although that may sound awful, the reality is, life is indeed burdensome for most of us. This burden or stress can become overwhelming for many. In extreme cases, suicide and depression, or dependence on drugs and alcohol may occur. In milder cases, overeating and obesity, or withdrawal and physical decline may develop. The templates imprinted within our brains during our youth or infancy represent the basic instincts created within our minds that we rely on to deal with these daily stresses. Our judgment however is not always based on sound advice and this can lead to poor decision making. This can be avoided by simply slowing down the process.

It should not be acceptable for us to rely on unconscious memories from our youth to make decisions for us as adults. We, as adults, need to develop an educated decision-making process so that we do not rush to judgment. Therefore, it is necessary to gather information and allow the adult brain to examine and decide, based on the present, how we will proceed. Once this is accomplished, through proper prospective, the scenarios described previously can and will be overcome. This is the prospective that can be recaptured only through Dimensionality.

Although most people will agree that mental stress brought on by life and its challenges can eventually express itself in a physical form. Few of us can identify what these stresses are and how they affect our lives, let alone comprehend the solution to the problem. Possibly the answer may lie in the fact that we as a society perceive stress as a vulnerability of character and an outside influence which affects our lives as apposed to the internal struggle that we ourselves have created.

For most of us it becomes difficult to accept stress as a diagnosis for our ailments. The last thing you want to hear from your physician is that your symptoms are due to stress. It makes us feel mentally vulnerable or weak as individuals, plus there is no pill to cure it, ultimately the reason we went to the physician in the first place. In addition, because we choose to believe that stress is an outside influence, we also tend to believe that a vacation or avoidance of the source will cure it. The truth however is that the stress is not the result of an outside source but rather a result of our interpretation or reaction to this outside influence. Simply, it is our own mental perception of the situation.

When a person has finally incorporated Dimensionality into their lives they will have a clearer perception of themselves. These individuals' exude confidence and express security in their thinking. When challenged with complicated tasks, these individuals will address such problems head on and formulate a solution. The task will be completed to the individuals' personal level of satisfaction. The challenge will have been dealt with and is therefore no longer a potential source of stress. On the other hand, individuals' who do not possess Dimensionality in their lives view themselves as inadequate, uncertain and by nature are procrastinators. In the worst cases, such people cannot complete even the simplest tasks. In-turn these unaddressed or incomplete items or tasks represent unfinished business, and thus, become added baggage, burdens or stressors for that individual.

In conclusion, we create our own stress based on the decisions we make. Whether we stop to think, procrastinate, or rush to judgment, we make our own choices. However, in many cases the daily decisions we make are really predetermined by templates laid down in our brains long ago. These templates can serve to influence our lives in a negative fashion everyday. Yet, we do not revisit these decisions to try and rethink and correct the consequences they have produced. Believe me when I tell you that there are reasons why people over eat, there are

reasons individuals hate their jobs, there are reasons why couples experience marital dissatisfaction and so on. We need to ask ourselves the
question so we can define the answer!

# *Dimensionality*

**-Take responsibility.**

> -It's your life!

**-We influence all things that matter.**

> -Our Perceptions.
> -How we feel.
> -How we act.
> -How we live.
> -It makes us who we are, or who we are not.

**-Reevaluate what is important to you.**

> -Commit to positive change.
> -Change your life for yourself and your family
> -You are a reflection of Humanity.
> -Prospective will keep you healthy.
> -Prospective can heal you.
> -Prospective can and will save your life.

# CHAPTER 10

▼

# WHAT JUST HAPPENED?

This chapter is included, in an effort, to provide moral support. The fact that the study of aging and the elderly is in its infancy, implies that there will be much indecision and many speed bumps along the way. Obviously, there is much yet to be learned before being offered a guarantee of aging successfully. Then again, there are few guarantees in life.

In addition, no matter how hard you work, things can and will go wrong, Murphy's Law is indeed a real phenomena. The functions of daily living are in many ways nothing more or less than statistical probabilities. Every time you cross a busy intersection there is a possibility that you might be run down by oncoming traffic. The simplest daily tasks carry with them the potential for disastrous consequences. Therefore, my constant daunting pessimistic reminder to all of you, expect the unexpected, because eventually it happens.

Obviously, the same holds true for the process of aging. Even if you follow the BHS Factor religiously, some things, at least for the time being, are just inevitable as we age. Hair will fallout and be lost from the usual places and grow profusely from unusual spaces. Wrinkles, dimples, and barnacle-like growths will find their way on to your persona. In addition, taste, sight, and sound can be expected to diminish.

Our memories may become nothing more than history, and our libidos just shrunken, wilted dreams. A variable smorgasbord of events that represent the pubescence stages of old age.

This potential list of changes we might expect with aging is obviously abbreviated. The purpose of this book is to be supportive and up lifting, while providing hope for the future. I certainly don't want to discourage or depress you before you even get started. So, as consolation, I offer you this, on that fateful day when you look in the mirror and think, "what the hell just happened?" I am confident that you will be able to take solace in your position. You will have had an advantage over all the others for having read this book.

The BHS Factor will have actually slowed your aging process. On this, so called, "day of reckoning," you will inevitably realize that you have faired better than the rest. Although this particular day may not be preventable, it will have been delayed in relation to the norm. The fact is, while this experience may occur on your ninetieth birthday, your counterpart will have undergone this experience at the age of seventy. Take solace in the fact that you are still alive and have maintained your independence. You will have surpassed the limits of current expectations and arrived there in a healthier, independent, and self sustained condition. You will have "bucked the system," and that is the premise of this book.

All indications suggest, the quicker you get started, the better off you will be in the long run. We as human beings have an inherent tendency towards self preservation. The BHS Factor provides just that, an opportunity for self preservation, the possibility to live longer without disability, the type of disability that strips us of our independence. If you know someone, or are yourself, in a position of caring for a parent or elderly loved one with physical and or mental limitations, you have obviously witnessed for yourself the devastation such conditions can bring.

I am confident those of you who are witnesses to such tragedy will join me in utilizing the BHS Factor for yourselves. The program is not strict and overly structured. It can be implemented at your pace, and is easy to do. Start walking and eliminate fats from your diets, you will lose weight, increase muscle tone and flexibility, and have initiated a new chapter in your life. Try loving yourself, stop taking yourself for granted and realize your true worth to yourself, your family and your community. You will be astonished by what you can accomplish by simply changing your mindset or perception. These changes will aid you to further incorporate future changes on a weekly or monthly basis. You will be able to add or delete from this program as you wish. You can create a program as structured or unstructured as you like. Just get started, because any and all improvement is positive, and more importantly, long lasting.

# Endnotes

1. Kane RL, Ouslander JG, Abrass IB, et al: The Elderly Patient: Demography and Epidemiology, in: Essentials of Clinical Geriatrics. New York City, McGraw-Hill 3rd Edition, 1994.

2. Chart Book on Trends in the Health of Americans: Health, United States, 2004; 20-21.

3. U.S. Bureau of Census, 1950 and 2000 Decennial Censuses: Health, United States, 2004; 153.

4. U.S. Bureau of Census, 2050 Interim Population Projections: Health, United States, 2004.

5. Chart Book on Trends in the Health of Americans: Health, United States, 2004; 21.

6. Centers for Medicare and Medicaid Services: Medicare Current Beneficiary Survey, Access to Care Files, United States, 2004.

7. Center for Disease Control and Prevention, National Center for Health Statistics: National Vital Statistics System, United States, 2004.

8. Kane RL, Ouslander JG, Abrass IB, et al: The Elderly Patient: Demography and Epidemiology, in: *Essentials of Clinical Geriatrics.* New York City, McGraw-Hill 3rd Edition, 1994.

9. A Long, Healthy Life: An Increasingly Common Phenomenon, *Live Longer Live Better.* The Readers Digest Association, Inc., New York, 1995.

10. National Center for Chronic Disease Prevention and Health Promotion: Chronic Disease Prevention; Chronic Disease Overview, (www.cdc.gov/nccdphp/overview.htm), 2005.

11. Chart Book on Trends in the Health of Americans: Health, United States, 2004; 26.

12. King MB, et al: Falls: The Principles of Geriatric Medicine and Gerontology. New York City, McGraw Hill Professional, 2003.

13. American Academy of Family Physicians: Metabolic Syndrome, Peer-Reviewed Bulletin; Vol.4/Number 2, 2005.

14. Hamer AM, The Geriatric Reporter: The Role of Cholinergic Function in Managing Disease Progression in Alzheimer's disease, Geriatric Times, April 2004.

15. Chart Book on Trends in the Health of Americans: Health and Poverty, United States, 2004; 40-42.

978-0-595-40312-7
0-595-40312-3